Computations in Nutrition: A guide for health care workers

1st Edition

by

Donnette Wright-Myrie

Phd candidate, MSc, BSc, RN

Affiliate: The University of the West Indies, Mona

Computations in Nutrition: A guide for health care workers

Copyright © 2018 by Donette Myrie, Msc, Bsc, RN
All rights reserved. This book or any portion thereof may not be reproduced or used in any manner whatsoever without the express written permission of the publisher except for the use of brief quotations in a book review.

Printed in the United States of America

ISBN 9781718692541

For more information on pricing, research or mass purchase contact the author at:

The University of the West Indies, Mona
The UWI School of Nursing, Mona
9 Gibraltar Camp Way, Mona, Kingston 7, Jamaica, WI.
Email: donnette.wright02@uwimona.edu.jm
Book Interior Design done by Kevan Ferguson
Wright-Myrie, Donnette. Computations in Nutrition: A guide for health care workers

Createspace Publishing
ISBN 9781718692541
1.Medical books—Nursing—Calculations and Computations. 2. Science and Technology — Nutrition Calculations. 3. Non-fiction—Math.

First Edition: May 2018

14 13 12 11 10 / 10 9 8 7 6 5 4 3 2 1

BeOne Foundation For Transformational Leadership

BeOne is about creating creators for family owned businesses.

BeOne means being undivided and one with life, one with nature and one with all creation.

BeOne is a place to go beyond the current construct and explore an intelligence beyond intellect. BeOne builds 10x foundations for businesses.

Creationist Methodology can be applied to solve almost any problem. But our minds and therefore our problems are often messy and complex—and need to be tackled with simplicity. That's where BeOne approach comes in. Enabling a person with BeOne's tools and methods often results in an instant transformation. A newfound construct transforms how people think, value and believe about themselves and their ability to have an impact on the world.

BeOne's impact can be seen in a variety of ways: within people themselves, on the businesses, in families, in nation building and in the world at large.

More details can be found at www.thebeone.com

About The Author

Chetan Walia is recognized by the corporate world as an educator, a consultant. He has a celebrated career spanning two decades in creating change and transformation for businesses across industries.

He has partnered with many International small and large companies. His principles and methodologies have been applied in almost every area of human endeavor from industry to education to the social sector.

Chetan Walia is the Chief Executive Officer at BeOne.

You can contact the author through the BeOne website – www.thebeone.com

This page was intentionally left blank.

TABLE OF CONTENTS

Revision of Conversion..........................1

Chapter 1: Body Mass Index

    Introduction...............................2
    Computation...............................2
    Classifications............................3
    Limitations................................4
    Practice Questions.........................5
    References.................................5

Chapter 2: Energy Computations: Physical Activity

    Introduction...............................6
    Computation................................7
    Limitations................................8
    Practice Questions.........................9
    References.............................9-10

Chapter 3: Energy Requirements

    Introduction..............................11
    Practice Questions.....................12-13
    References................................14

Chapter 4: Energy Computations: Physical Activity

Introduction.................................15
Computation using BMR and PAL......16
Atwater Factors...........................16
Computation using Atwater factors....16
Practice Questions....................16-17
References..............................18-19

Chapter 5: Malnutrition Universal Screening Tool

Introduction.................................20
Steps of MUST........................21-23
Limitations..............................23-24
Practice Questions....................24-25
References.................................26

Chapter 6: Waist Hip Ratio

Introduction.................................27
Interpretations............................28
Computation................................28
Practice Questions....................29-30
References..............................30-31

TABLE OF CONTENTS

Chapter 7: Calculating energy requirements for Intravenous administration

Introduction..............................32
Computation.........................33-34
Notes..34
Practice Questions.......................35
References................................36

Chapter 8: Ideal Body Weight

Introduction..............................37
Predictions...........................38-39
Computations.......................38-39
Practice Questions.......................40
References................................41

ANSWER SHEET 42-53

Computations in Nutrition: A guide for health care workers

The first step in computing is understanding how to convert. Here is a summary conversion table between common imperial and metric units.

Table 1: Conversion between imperial and metric units

Large Unit	Small Unit
1 inch	2.54 cm
1 kg	2.2 lbs
1 foot	12 inches
1 kcal	4.184 kj
1 m	100 cm
1 lb	16 ounces

Note: When converting between units remember; from a larger unit to a smaller unit, you multiply & from a smaller to a larger unit, you divide.

Chapter 1

Body Mass Index

Body mass index (BMI) is important in assessing health status and serves as a valuable tool to health care workers. It was reported that an increase of 1 standard deviation in BMI was associated with 2·63–3·70 mmHg increase in systolic blood pressure (SBP) in children. Current evidence provides data that there are concordant Increases in the obesity rates and chronic disease prevalence, particularly hypertension (Zou, Wang, Dong, Li, & Ma, 2016). The computation is simple and can be done using either metric or imperial methodology.

The Metric computation formula is:

$$\text{Weight (kg)} / \text{Height (m}^2)$$

Here is an example of how the formula is applied:
John weighs 5 kg and is 0.5 m tall. What is his BMI?

Answer.
BMI= 5 (kg)/0 .5 (m) x .5 (m)
= 5(kg)/ 0.25 (m²)
= 20kg/m²

$$\text{The Imperial computation formula is:} \\ \text{Weight (lbs)} \div \text{Height}$$

Here is an example of how the formula is applied:
Peter weighs 180 lbs and is six feet tall. Calculate his BMI using the imperial formula?

Answer
=180 lbs/ (72 [in] x 72 [in]) x 703
[N.B. 6 feet= 72 inches; i.e. 6 x 12= 72]
= 180/5184 x 703
= 0.0347 x 703
=24.39 lbs/inches^2

BMI Classifications

For adults 20 years and older BMI may be interpreted based on WHO weight standards (see table 1).

Table 2: BMI Classifications

BMI	BMI Categorisation
Below 18.5	Underweight
18.5 – 24.9	Normal or Healthy Weight
25.0 – 29.9	Overweight
30.0 – 34.9	Obese Class 1
35.0 – 39.9	Obese Class 2
≥ 40.0	Obese Class 3/morbid obesity

Di Angelantonio, *et al.* (2016)

Interpretation of examples

Using the BMI classifications both John and Peter would be classified as having normal weight.

Limitations of BMI

Limitations of BMI include its significant underestimation of body fat in differing populations and incorrect classification of individuals who are muscular as overweight and obese (Nash, 2015).

Using the examples above complete the following

1. A man, height 1.60m, weight 70kg
2. A woman, height 1.52m, weight 50kg
3. A woman, height 1.55m, weight 48kg
4. A woman, height 1.63m, weight 100kg
5. A man, height 1.78m, weight 93kg
6. A man, height 1.63m, weight 54kg
7. A man, height 1.80m, weight 113kg
8. A woman, height 1.65m, weight 49kg
9. A woman, height 1.52m, weight 97kg
10. A man, height 1.83m, weight 61kg
11. A man, height 5 feet 8 inches, weight 155 lbs
12. A woman, height 5 feet 4 inches, weight 130 lbs
13. A woman, height 5 feet 7.5 inches, weight 147 lbs
14. A woman, height 5 feet 3 inches, weight 128 lbs
15. A man, height 5 feet 9 inches, weight 162 lbs
16. A man, height 5 feet 8 inches, weight 154 lbs
17. A man, height 5 feet 8.5 inches, weight 120 lbs
18. A woman, height 5 feet 5 inches, weight 138 lbs
19. A woman, height 5 feet 6 inches, weight 144 lbs
20. A man, height 5 feet 10 inches, weight 167 lbs

See answers on *page 40 and 41*

References

CDC. (2017). About adult BMI. Retrieved from http://www.cdc.gov/healthyweight/assessing/bmi/adult_bmi/index.html

Di Angelantonio, E., Bhupathiraju, S. N., Wormser, D., Gao, P., Kaptoge, S., de Gonzalez, A. B., ... & Lewington, S. (2016). Body-mass index and all-cause mortality: Individual-participant-data meta-analysis of 239 prospective studies in four continents. *The Lancet, 388*(10046), 776-786.

Nash, M. S. (2015). Editorial Note on: Optimal scaling of weight and waist circumference to height for adiposity and cardiovascular disease risk in individuals with spinal cord injury. Retrieved from https://www.nature.com/articles/sc2014176

Zou, Z. Y., Wang, S., Dong, B., Li, X. H., & Ma, J. (2016). The importance of blood lipids in the association between BMI and blood pressure among Chinese overweight and obese children. *British Journal of Nutrition, 116*(1), 45-51.

Chapter 2
Energy Requirements

Basal metabolic rate represents the baseline energy cost of maintaining body systems and processes critical to sustaining life (Auer, Salin, Rudolf, Anderson, & Metcalfe, 2015). Resting metabolic rate (RMR) which is similar to BMR, but occurs at steady homeostatic conditions, is described as the largest component of total energy needs and expenditure. It is strongly impacted by lean body mass and to a smaller extent by fat mass, age, and sex which account for a combined 7–9% of the variance in RMR (McNeil *et al*, 2017). This is important to health care workers because it may be used to determine clients' needs and to help prevent chronic diseases. There are several formulae that can be used to compute BMR, one formula that is used often in literature is the Harris-Benedict Formula, and it is described below.

The Harris-Benedict Formula

For women: BMR = 655 + (9.6 x weight in kilos) + (1.8 x height in cm) − (4.7 x age in years)

For men: BMR = 665 + (13.7 x weight in kilos) + (5 x height in cm) − (6.8 x age in years)

Worked Examples

Example 1: 20 year old Shauna weighs 54kg, and is 1.2 m tall. Calculate her BMR.

Answer:

BMR = 655+ (9.6 x 54) + (1.8 x 120) – (4.7 x 20)
= 655+ (518.4) + (216) - (94)
= 1389.4-94
= 1295.4 Kcal

Example 2: 22 year old Shaun weighs 68kg, and is 1.6 m tall. Calculate his BMR.

Answer

BMR = 66 + (13.7 x 68) + (5 x 160) – (6.8 x 22)
= 66 + (931.6) + (800) – (149.6)
= 1797.6-149.6
= 1648 Kcal

Limitations of Harris Benedict equation

Though resting energy expenditure can be measured by calorimetry, direct and indirect, it is most often estimated by equations including the Harris Benedict formula. This equation has been described in contemporary literature as the most accurate prediction of energy needs. Nevertheless, it has been criticized has having low predictivity in thermally injured clients and clients with gastric oncology due to variability in their metabolism (Amirkalali, Hosseini, Heshmat, & Larijani, 2008). Other contemporary evidence suggests that in patients with significant illnesses, the altered metabolic milieu increases REE and renders the precision of the formula indefinite (Hashemian, *et al.*, 2017).

Using the examples above compute the following questions:

1. 21 year old female weighs 52 kg, and is 128 cm tall. Calculate her BMR.
2. 23 year old male weighs 65 kg, and is 1.63 m tall. Calculate his BMR.
3. 37 year old female weighs 48 kg, and is 132 cm tall. Calculate her BMR.
4. 43 year old male weighs 69 kg, and is 1.58 m tall. Calculate his BMR.
5. 30 year old female weighs 54 kg, and is 1.4 m tall. Calculate her BMR.

Questions (cont'd)

6. 33 year old male weighs 74 kg, and is 1.68 m tall. Calculate his BMR.
7. 35 year old female weighs 50 kg, and is 125 cm tall. Calculate her BMR.
8. 27 year old male weighs 55 kg, and is 1.58 m tall. Calculate his BMR.
9. 24 year old female weighs 43 kg, and is 118 cm tall. Calculate her BMR.
10. 50 year old male weighs 66 kg, and is 1.61 m tall. Calculate his BMR.

See answer on *pages 41 and 42.*

References

Amirkalali, B., Hosseini, S., Heshmat, R., & Larijani, B. (2008). Comparison of Harris Benedict and Mifflin-ST Jeor equations with indirect calorimetry in evaluating resting energy expenditure. *Indian Journal of Medical Sciences*, 62(7), 283.

Auer, S. K., Salin, K., Rudolf, A. M., Anderson, G. J., & Metcalfe, N. B. (2015). Flexibility in metabolic rate confers a growth advantage under changing food availability. *Journal of Animal Ecology*, *84*(5), 1405-1411.

Hashemian, S. M., Martindale, R. G., Jamaati, H., Amirsavadkouhi, A., Azer, S. M., Shadnoush, M., ... & Mahmoodpoor, A. (2017). An Iranian Consensus Document for Nutrition in Critically Ill Patients, Recommendations and Initial Steps toward Regional Guidelines. *Tanaffos*, 16(2), 89.

McNeil, J., Lamothe, G., Cameron, J. D., Riou, M. È., Cadieux, S., Lafrenière, J. ... & Doucet, É. (2017). Investigating predictors of eating: is resting metabolic rate really the strongest proxy of energy intake?. *The American Journal of Clinical Nutrition*, *106*(5), 1206-1212.

Chapter 3
Energy Computations: Physical Activity

Physical activity is defined as any functional movement produced by skeletal muscles that results in energy expenditure. The energy expenditure may be measured in kilocalories or kilojoules (Locke *et al*, 2015; Caspersen, Powell, & Christenson, 1985). The examination of the components of energy expenditure (EE) including estimating physical activity (PA) in humans is important in stemming global non-communicable diseases (Hills, Mokhtar, & Byrne, 2014). This concept can be computed using the formula outlined below.

$$PAL = TDEE \div BMR$$
[TDEE- Total Daily Energy Expenditure]

If Sharon's total energy expenditure for the last 24 hours is 1836.5 Kcal and her BMR is 1479.8 Kcal. What is her PAL? Categorise her PAL.

Answer.

PAL = TDEE ÷ BMR
= 1836.5/1479.8
= 1.24

PAL category: Sedentary

Physical activity levels can be interpreted based on the table below

Table 3: Physical Activity Classifications

CATERGORY	PAL	DESCRIPTION
SEDENTARY	1.2	little or no exercise, desk job
LIGHTLY ACTIVE	1.375	light exercise/sports 1-3 days/wk
MODERATELY ACTIVE	1.55	moderate exercise/sports 3-5 days/wk
VERY ACTIVE	1.725	hard exercise/sports 6-7 days/wk
EXTRA ACTIVE	1.9	hard daily exercise/sports & physical job or 2X day training, marathon, football camp, contest, etc.

(Westerterp, 2013).

Using the examples above compute the following questions:

1. What is the PAL of an individual who has total energy expenditure for the last 24 hours is 1850 Kcal and her BMR is 1480 Kcal? Categorise the person's PAL.
2. What is the PAL of an individual who has total energy expenditure for the last 24 hours is 1920 Kcal and her BMR is 1525 Kcal? Categorise the person's PAL.
3. What is the PAL of an individual who has total energy expenditure for the last 24 hours is 1657.5 Kcal and her BMR is 1336.5 Kcal? Categorise the person's PAL.

5. What is the PAL of an individual who has total energy expenditure for the last 24 hours is 2268 Kcal and her BMR is 1748.2 Kcal? Categorise the person's PAL.
6. What is the PAL of an individual who has total energy expenditure for the last 24 hours is 2300 Kcal and her BMR is 1689 Kcal? Categorise the person's PAL.
7. What is the PAL of an individual who has total energy expenditure for the last 24 hours is 1961 Kcal and her BMR is 1265 Kcal? Categorise the person's PAL.
8. What is the PAL of an individual who has total energy expenditure for the last 24 hours is 1960 Kcal and her BMR is 1400 Kcal? Categorise the person's PAL.
9. What is the PAL of an individual who has total energy expenditure for the last 24 hours is 2250 Kcal and her BMR is 1410 Kcal? Categorise the person's PAL.
10. What is the PAL of an individual who has total energy expenditure for the last 24 hours is 1800 Kcal and her BMR is 1280 Kcal? Categorise the person's PAL.
11. What is the PAL of an individual who has total energy expenditure for the last 24 hours is 1750 Kcal and her BMR is 1400 Kcal? Categorise the person's PAL.

See answers on *page 42 and 43*

References

Caspersen, C. J., Powell, K. E., & Christenson, G. M. (1985). Physical activity, exercise, and physical fitness: definitions and distinctions for health-related research. *Public Health Reports, 100*(2), 126.

Hills, A. P., Mokhtar, N., & Byrne, N. M. (2014). Assessment of physical activity and energy expenditure: an overview of objective measures. *Frontiers in Nutrition, 1*, 5.

Locke, A. E., Kahali, B., Berndt, S. I., Justice, A. E., Pers, T. H., Day, F. R., ... & Croteau-Chonka, D. C. (2015). Genetic studies of body mass index yield new insights for obesity biology. *Nature, 518*(7538), 197.

Westerterp, K. R. (2013). Physical activity and physical activity induced energy expenditure in humans: measurement, determinants, and effects. *Frontiers in Physiology, 4*, 90.

Chapter 4
Calculating Total Energy Intake

Dietary intake patterns are integral to the incidence of global chronic disease burden (Imamura, *et al*, 2015). Computing energy intake may assist in managing the development and maintenance of obesity and provide cues for health maintenance (Blundell, *et al*, 2015). There are several strategies used to estimate and determine total energy intake and are useful in preventing chronic diseases. Atwater factors are important in manual computations of gross chemical energy. Its application is useful in determining the quantity of chemical energy trapped in food based on the relative mass of the product (Sanghvi, *et al*, 2015; Acheson, *et al*, 1980). Total energy intake can be computed based on the mass of a macronutrient in a commodity while total energy requirement may be assessed by multiplying physical activity level by Basal Metabolic Rate. The formulae are demonstrated in the examples below.

> *Caloric Requirement* - BMR x PAL

Shari has a BMR of 1524 kcal/day and is moderately active. How many calories must she take in per day to meet her caloric requirements?

Answer
TER = BMR x PAL
TER = 1524Kcal*1.55
    = 2362.22 Kcal

Table 4: Atwater factors

Macronutrients and Alcohol	Energy contribution
Protein	4 kcal/g
Carbohydrate	4 kcal/g
Fat	9 kcal/g
Alcohol	7 kcal/g

Shari consumes a product that reads 5 grams per serving. The persons eats 12.5 grams. The label reads 10 g carbohydrates, 5 grams protein and 4 grams fat per serving. What is the total energy that the person consumes?

Answer.
Total serving consumed = 12.5g/5g = 2.5 servings

Carbohydrates = 10 g x 2.5　　　*Fats* = 4 g x 2.5
　　　　　　　= 25 x 4 Kcal/g　　　　　= 10 x 9 Kcal
　　　　　　　(Atwater factor)　　　　(Atwater factor)
　　　　　　　= 100 Kcal　　　　　　　= 90 Kcal

Proteins　　= 5 g x 2.5
　　　　　　= 12.5 x 4 Kcal/g
　　　　　　(Atwater factor)
　　　　　　= 50 Kcal

Total energy = 100+50+90 = 240 Kcal

Using the examples above compute the following questions:

1. A client consumes a juice box with 1.5 servings as the total content. Each serving contains 22 g of carbohydrates; and 16 g of protein consumed. What is the client's TEI?
2. What is the total energy in food with the following macronutrient composition: 5 g alcohol; 12.5 g carbohydrate; 17 g protein and 3g fat?
3. How much energy does an individual receive if he consumes 3.5 servings of a product which has 28 g of carbohydrate, 14 g of fat and 18.5 g of protein per serving?
4. Determine the TEI of a client who drinks 600 mls of a product that reads 250 mls per serving which has 10 g alcohol, 7 g carbohydrate and 30 g of protein per serving.
5. What is the energy contribution of a product that has 15g of carbohydrate, 8 g of protein and 4 grams of fat per serving if the client has 5 servings?
6. What is the energy contribution of a product that has 13 g of carbohydrate, 64 g of protein and 8 g of fat, if a client has 2 servings?
7. A client consumes a 750 ml bottle of a beverage which reads 300 mls per serving. It has 40 g Carbs, 12 g fat and 28 g of alcohol per serving. What is the TEI of the client who consumes this beverage?

> *Questions (cont'd)*
>
> 8. What is the total energy in food with the following macronutrient composition: 30 g carbohydrate, 17 g protein and 5 g of fat?
> 9. How much energy does a client receive from 4 servings of a product which has 11.5 g of carbohydrate, 14 g of protein and 10 g of fat?
> 10. Determine the total energy a client receives if he consumes 2.5 servings of a product which has 15 g of carbohydrates, 32 g of protein and 16 g fat

See answers on *pages 44 and 45*.

References

Acheson, K. J., Campbell, I. T., Edholm, O. G., Miller, D. S., & Stock, M. J. (1980). The measurement of food and energy intake in man—an evaluation of some techniques. *The American Journal of Clinical Nutrition, 33*(5), 1147-1154.

Blundell, J. E., Finlayson, G., Gibbons, C., Caudwell, P., & Hopkins, M. (2015). The biology of appetite control: do resting metabolic rate and fat-free mass drive energy intake?. *Physiology & Behavior, 152*, 473-478.

Imamura, F., Micha, R., Khatibzadeh, S., Fahimi, S., Shi, P., Powles, J., ... & Global Burden of Diseases Nutrition and Chronic Diseases Expert Group (NutriCoDE. (2015).

Dietary quality among men and women in 187 countries in 1990 and 2010: a systematic assessment. *The Lancet Global Health*, *3*(3), e132-e142.

Sanghvi, A., Redman, L. M., Martin, C. K., Ravussin, E., & Hall, K. D. (2015). Validation of an inexpensive and accurate mathematical method to measure long-term changes in free-living energy intake, 2. *The American Journal of Clinical Nutrition*, *102*(2), 353-358.

Chapter 5
Malnutrition Universal Screening Tool (M.U.S.T.)

The 'Malnutrition Universal Screening Tool' ('M.U.S.T.') was created to assist in the categorisation of adults who are underweight and at risk of malnutrition, as well as those who are obese. It was not designed to detect deficiencies in or excessive intakes of vitamins and minerals (Todorovic, Russell, Stratton, Ward, & Elia, 2003). It is one of many public health tools that are useful in assessing at risk populations and involves simple computations of three nutritional parameters; BMI, unplanned weight loss, and intake or disease. M.U.S.T has been described as being very useful in acute diseases but has limitations in detecting nutritional risk in the institutionalized elderly population (Diekmann, *et al*, 2013). The tool has been validated in the oncology population and found to be useful in antedating detailed nutritional assessment and predicting nutritional risk based on weight loss over 3 to 6 months (Boléo-Tomé, Monteiro-Grillo, Camilo, & Ravasco, 2012).

The tool is used in a stepwise process demonstrated in the example below.

Step 1. Compute BMI and then assign a score of 0 to 2 based on results

BMI Score
0= > 20
1= 18.5 -20.0
2=< 18.5

Step 2. Compute unplanned weight loss by subtracting current weight from usual weight, using result as a percent of usual weight. Assign scores of 0 to 2 to percent weight loss

Unplanned weight loss score
        0=<5%
        1= 5-10%
        2=>10%

Step 3. Acute disease score: If there is an acute pathophysiological or psychological state, and there has been negligible or no nutritional intake or likelihood of no intake for more than 5 days, there is a high probability of nutritional risk (Todorovic, *et al*, 2003).

Scores of 2 or 0 are assigned in this category, where 2 = none or negligible intake for >5 days, 0 = no impairments to intake or impairments lasting less than 5 days

Step 4. Add the scores in steps 1 to 3 to calculate overall risk of malnutrition and categorize the risk
    0 = low risk: routine clinical care
    1 = medium risk: observe
    2 or more= high risk: treat

Example 1: James is 21 years old and weighed 45kg last month and now weighs 41 kg. He is 155 cm tall. He has had little intake for the 2 weeks and has stage 3 cancer. Calculate his MUST score and classify him.

Step 1

BMI = 41/1.55 x 1.55
= 41/2.4025
=17.07kg/m^2

BMI score= 2 (BMI less than 18.5)

Step 2

Percentage weight loss:
Current percentage of usual weight = 45 - 41 = 4 kg
Percentage weight loss = 4/45 x 100= 8.89 %
Weight loss score= 1 (5-10%)

Step 3

Disease score = 2 (intake minimal for more than 5 days)

Step 4: Compute the overall score

2 (BMI score) + 1 (Weight loss score) + 2 (Disease score)
Total score = 5

Classification
High Risk-Treat

Note Breifly that:
1. Scores are always whole numbers;
2. Overall scores range from 0 to 6;
3. Lower scores are related to lower nutritional risk,
4. And higher scores are associated with greater risk of undernutrition

Limitations of M.U.S.T.

Though useful in assessing hospitalized patients progress and nutritional risk. The tool's use is contingent on the knowledge, skill and expertise of the health care workers. Contemporary evidence identify that the use of the MUST should be complimented with an understanding of physical and psychological factors that could cause poor dietary intake and increase nutritional risk (Robertson, 2015).

Moreover the authors suggested that *"to holistically care for a patient the use of a tool, such as MUST, needs to be a framework from which to work; signposting a need not suggesting a solution. Each patient's contributing factors to their need is going to be different even if the need is the same"* (p. 4).

Using the example above compute the following

1. A client weighed 52kg last month and now weighs 49.5 kg. He is 1.61 m tall. He has had little intake for the 2 days. Calculate his MUST score and classify him.
2. A client weighed 63 kg last month and now weighs 64.3 kg. He is 166 cm tall. He has had no intake for the 6 days. Calculate his MUST score and classify him
3. A client weighed 48 kg last month and now weighs 46.2 kg. He is 1.58 m tall. He has had little intake for the 4 days. Calculate his MUST score and classify him
4. A client weighed 61 kg last month and now weighs 60.4 kg. He is 1.75 m tall. He has had little intake for the 3 days. Calculate his MUST score and classify him

Questions(cont'd)

5. A client weighed 55kg last month and now weighs 52.6 kg. He is 163.5 cm tall. He has had little intake for the 4 days. Calculate his MUST score and classify him
6. A client weighed 60 kg last month and now weighs 57 kg. He is 1.65 m tall. He has had little intake for the 1 day. Calculate his MUST score and classify him
7. A client weighed 65kg last month and now weighs 63.5 kg. He is 172 cm tall. He has had little intake for the 3 days. Calculate his MUST score and classify him
8. A client weighed 68kg last month and now weighs 66.5 kg. He is 1.73 m tall. He has had little intake for the 6 days. Calculate his MUST score and classify him
9. A client weighed 55kg last month and now weighs 53 kg. He is 162 cm tall. He has had little intake for the 2 days. Calculate his MUST score and classify him
10. A client weighed 48kg last month and now weighs 47 kg. He is 158 cm tall. He has had little intake for the 4 days. Calculate his MUST score and classify him

See answers on *pages 48 and 49*

References

Boléo-Tomé, C., Monteiro-Grillo, I., Camilo, M., & Ravasco, P. (2012). Validation of the malnutrition universal screening tool (MUST) in cancer. *British Journal of Nutrition*, 108(2), 343-348.-348.

Diekmann, R., Winning, K., Uter, W., Kaiser, M. J., Sieber, C., Volkert, D., & Bauer, J. M. (2013). Screening for malnutrition among nursing home residents—a comparative analysis of the Mini Nutritional Assessment, the Nutritional Risk Screening, and the Malnutrition Universal Screening Tool. *The Journal of Nutrition, Health & Aging*, 17(4), 326-331.

Robertson, L. (2015). Evaluating the Malnutrition Universal Screening Tool as a holistic client assessment and critically appraising the evidence relating to meeting the essential nutritional needs of a patient. *Health Sciences*, 1(12), 1-9.

Todorovic, V., Russell, C., Stratton, R., Ward, J., & Elia, M. (2003). The 'MUST' explanatory booklet: a guide to the 'Malnutrition Universal Screening Tool' ('MUST') for adults. *Redditch: British Association for Parenteral and Enteral Nutrition (BAPEN)*.

Chapter 6
Waist Hip Ratio

There is a strong link between central adiposity and chronic non-communicable diseases particularly diabetes especially in the African- American population. Among the multiple measures of central adiposity (BMI), waist circumference (WC), hip circumference (HC), waist–hip-ratio (WHR) and waist–height-ratio (WHtR), particular measures such as WC was determined to be the best predictor of chronic illnesses and to some extent WHtR, however BMI and WHR were determined to be valuable but less effective (Mbanya, Kengne, Mbanya, & Akhtar, 2015). Current evidence describes BMI and WC as the best surrogates of visceral adiposity index but identify that WHR is an acceptable surrogate of visceral adiposity index (Borruel, *et al.,* 2014). Contemporary literature also provides explanations as to the validity and sensitivity of WHR and WC as measures of central adiposity and predictors of cardiovascular risk. Moreover, The World Health Organization (2011) proposes that theoretically, differences in measurements protocols across studies could be responsible for variations in the sensitivity of the index that is the predicted association of these measures with risk factors, or disease or mortality outcomes. Nevertheless, the Organization recognizes WHR as an acceptable standard for examining cardiovascular risk.
WHR is computed by diving WC by HC
Waist circumference (unit)/hip circumference (unit)

Note briefly that:
1. Units must be the same
2. Parameters are always computed in accurate anatomical positions with waist above hip
3. WHR is the ratio of the circumference of the waist to that of the hip
4. The result of the computation is devoid of a unit (i.e. unitless).

Interpretations

WHO STEPS states that abdominal obesity is defined as a waist–hip ratio above 0.90 for males and above 0.85 for females as increased cardiovascular risk in the African population and at higher levels for European and Asian populations (WHO, 2011).

Example 1: Fay has a waist circumference of 32 cm and a hip circumference of 14.96 inches. What is her WHR and WHO recommendations for her?

WHR = WC/HC in same unit

Convert HC- cm = 14.96 in x 2.54cm/ 1 in
 = 38 cm

Divide WC by HC = 32/38
 = 0.84

Low cardiovascular risk (normal)

Using the example above compute the following questions:

1. A client has a waist circumference of 71 cm and a hip circumference of 34 inches. What is **her** WHR and WHO recommendations for her?
2. A client has a waist circumference of 74 cm and a hip circumference of 36.8 cm. What is **her** WHR and WHO recommendations for her?
3. A client a waist circumference of 35 inches and a hip circumference of 33 inches. What is **his** WHR and WHO recommendations for her?
4. A client a waist circumference of 34 inches and a hip circumference of 35.2 inches. What is her WHR and WHO recommendations for **her**?
5. A client a waist circumference of 42 inches and a hip circumference of 46 inches. What is her WHR and WHO recommendations for **his**?
6. A client a waist circumference of 79 cm and a hip circumference of 83 cm. What is her WHR and WHO recommendations for **her**?
7. A client a waist circumference of 73 cm and a hip circumference of 38.2 inches. What is her WHR and WHO recommendations for **his**?
8. A client a waist circumference of 38 inches and a hip circumference of 39.2 cm. What is her WHR and WHO recommendations for **her**?
9. A client a waist circumference of 42 inches and a hip circumference of 46 inches. What is her WHR and WHO recommendations for **his**?

Questions (cont'd)
10. A client a waist circumference of 70 cm and a hip circumference of 81 cm. What is her WHR and WHO recommendations for **her**?

See answers on *pages 48 and 49*

References

Borruel, S., Moltó, J. F., Alpañés, M., Fernández-Durán, E., Álvarez-Blasco, F., Luque-Ramírez, M., & Escobar-Morreale, H. F. (2014). Surrogate markers of visceral adiposity in young adults: waist circumference and body mass index are more accurate than waist hip ratio, model of adipose distribution and visceral adiposity index. *PloS one*, 9(12), e114112.

Mbanya, V. N., Kengne, A. P., Mbanya, J. C., & Akhtar, H. (2015). Body mass index, waist circumference, hip circumference, waist–hip-ratio and waist–height-ratio: Which is the better discriminator of prevalent screen-detected diabetes in a Cameroonian population?. *Diabetes Research and Clinical Practice*, 108(1), 23-30.

World Health Organization. (2011). Waist circumference and waist-hip ratio: report of a WHO expert consultation, Geneva, 8-11 December 2008.

Chapter 7
Calculating Energy Intake from Intravenous Administration

Intravenous fluid administration is a treatment approach adopted to maintain or restore circulation to vital organs following loss of intravascular volume due to bleeding, plasma loss, or excessive external fluid and electrolyte loss, usually from the gastrointestinal (GI) tract, or severe internal losses (Padhi, Bullock & Stroud, 2013). Fluid requirements for adults are computed based on body weight and ranges from 1.5L to 3L while energy requirements are 25 to 35 kcal/kg/d dependent on the disease state of the individual (Flanagan, *et al*, 2012). Glucose content in intravenous fluids exists in many formulations including 5%, 10%, 20%, 25%, 50% and 70% preparations (Baxter Healthcare, 2014). Contemporary evidence points to the variability of the standards for determining energy contribution of intravenous solutions. The evidence proposes with glycerol included in lipid intravenous formulations energy yield for that lipid containing product was determined to be 10 rather than 9 kcal/g; some authors use 9 kcal per g for enteral fat and 10 kcal per g for parenteral fat. For carbohydrate (dextrose) some authors use 3.4 kcal per g because dextrose datasheets state that 1 g of dextrose contains 3.4 kcal, whereas others use the Atwater factor of 4 kcal per gram (Cormack, 2016). Manufacturers use 3.4 kcal/g as the energy contribution of dextrose.

Computations of energy in IV fluids are done as follows:

Nurse Joy is caring for an ill client. The client is ordered to 20% DW in 500 mls and prescribed 1L in 24 hours. How many calories is the client receiving daily? What volume of 20% fluid and how many bags of 20% DW fluid are needed to meet a requirement of 1600 kcal?

Volume of Dextrose in 500ml bag
= 20/100 x 500
= 100mls

$$If\ 1ml = 1g$$

Thus;
$$100mls\ dextrose = 100g\ dextrose$$

Number of calories provided by each bag of DW
= volume of dextrose per bag x 3.4 Kcal
= 100 x 3.4 Kcal = 340 Kcal

Number of calories in 1L
Conversion of L --> mLs
$$1L = 1000mls$$

Thus;
Number of bags in 1L
= 1000/ 500
= 2 bags

Computations of energy in IV fluids (cont'd)

If 340 Kcal = 1 bag (500 mLs)

Therefore;
  1L = 340 x 2
     = 680 kcal

Bags for 1600 kcal = 340 kcal in 500 mLs

Therefore;

Energy in 1ml = 340/500
             = 0.68 kcal per mil

1600 kcal = 1600 kcal/ 0.68 kcal x 1 ml
         = 1088 mLs

Hence;
The Number of bags needed = 1088 mLs/ 500 mLs x 1 bag
                            = 2.176 bags

Note briefly:

I. Atwater factor/ energy (kcal) per gram of carbohydrate for dextrose is 3.4 kcal/g
II. Percentage of carbohydrate in IV solution determines the mass of macronutrient consumed
III. 5% DW in 500 mls- means 5/100 * 500= 25 g Dextrose

Using the example above compute the following:

1. Compute the energy contribution for a client who received 1350 mls of 25% DW in 24 hours.
2. Compute the energy contribution for a client who received 1800 mls of 10% DW in 24 hours.
3. Compute the energy contribution for a client who received 2200 mls of 5% DW in 24 hours.
4. Compute the energy contribution for a client who received 3500 mls of 10% DW in 24 hours.
5. Compute the energy contribution for a client who received 2100 mls of 20% DW in 24 hours.
6. Compute the energy contribution for a client who received 1750 mls of 10% DW in 24 hours.
7. Compute the energy contribution for a client who received 3200 mls of 5% DW in 24 hours.
8. Compute the energy contribution for a client who received 1950 mls of 25% DW in 24 hours.
9. Compute the energy contribution for a client who received 1850 mls of 5% DW in 24 hours.
10. Compute the energy contribution for a client who received 950 mls of 50% DW in 24 hours.

See answers for questions in last chapter on *pages 49 and 50*

References

Baxter Healthcare, (2014). Glucose Intravenous Infusion, Viaflex bag: product information. Retrieved from http://www.baxterhealthcare.com.au/downloads/healthc are_professionals/cmi_pi/glucose%20IVI_pi.pdf

Cormack, B. E., Embleton, N. D., van Goudoever, J. B., Hay Jr, W. W., & Bloomfield, F. H. (2016). Comparing apples with apples: it is time for standardized reporting of neonatal nutrition and growth studies. *Pediatric Research*, 79(6), 810.

Flanagan, D., Fisher, T., Murray, M., Visvanathan, R., Charlton, K., Thesing, C., ... & Walther, K. (2012). Managing undernutrition in the elderly: Prevention is better than cure. *Australian Family Physician*, 41(9), 695.

Padhi, S., Bullock, I., Li, L., & Stroud, M. (2013). Intravenous fluid therapy for adults in hospital: summary of NICE guidance. *BMJ: British Medical Journal (Online)*, 347.

Chapter 8
Ideal Body Weight

Ideal body weight is an assessment and computational technique that can be used for health promotional purposes including the assessment of nutritional risk (Kammerer, Porter, Beekley, & Tichansky, 2015). Contemporary computations that adjust weight for height are used to estimate different nutritional and anthropometric states; underweight, overweight, and weight-associated health risks and mortality risk (Müller, 2016). Ideal body weight (IBW) is also considered as "healthy" weight and was defined according to its association with lowest mortality risk. In the last decade nutritional advances have been realised through the work of Hamwi, Devine and more recent work by Peterson and colleagues (Peterson, Thomas, Blackburn, & Heymsfield, 2016). The seminal work of computing ideal body weight was purposed with identifying desirable, targeted or ideal body weight. Throughout the past century, different IBW algorithms have been developed based on the general idea that height defines weight as a linear function (Müller, 2016). There are varying predictions and algorithms that can be used to determine ideal body weight, three of them are described below.

HAMWI'S PREDICTIONS (IMPERIAL UNITS)

For men: 106 lb for the first 5 ft; 6 lb for each inch over 5 ft ($\pm 10\%$)

For women: 100 lb for the first 5 ft; 5 lb for each inch over 5 ft (±10%)

HAMWI'S PREDICTION (METRIC UNITS)

Male = 48 kg for the first 152.4 cm + 1.1 kg for each additional cm (±10%)
Female = 45 kg for the first 152.4 cm + 0.9 kg for each additional cm (±10%)

Note briefly (N.B): Frame size can be estimated using wrist circumference, or elbow breadth measurement. More recently the WHO has come up with a formula for IBW

USING BMI

Males/Females = [**BMI**] 18.5 x (height in m^2)
[**BMI**] 24.9 x (height in m^2)

Example 1. A male client visits a health centre and reports that he is 5 feet 10 inches tall. Compute his ideal body weight using Hamwi Predictions Imperial and Metric and BMI predictions.

Hamwi IBW Imperial = 5 feet is 106 lbs
6 x 10 = 60lbs

Median weight = 106 + 60 = 166 lbs

10% value = 166 x 0.1 = 16.6lbs
Lower value   = 166-16.6
               = 149.4 lbs

Higher value = 166 + 16.6
= 182.6 lbs

IBW imperial weight range = 149.4 to 182.6 lbs

Hamwi IBW metric = convert height

5 x 12 = 60 + 10 = 70 inches x 2.54 = 177.8 cm
152.4 cm = 48 kg

Excess height = 177.8 - 152.4 = 25.4 cm
Add. Weight = 25.4 x 1.1 = 27.94 kg
Median weight = 48 + 27.94 = 75.94 kg

10% value = 75.94 x 0.1 = 7.59
Lower value = 75.94 - 7.59 = 68.35 kg
Higher value = 75.94 + 7.59 = 83.53 kg
IBW metric range = 68.35 to 83.53 kg

BMI predictions = squared height x 18.5 and 24.9

177.8 cm to m = 1.78 m
1.78 x 1.78 = 3.17
18.5 x 3.17 = 58.65
24.9 x 3.17 = 78.93

IBW BMI ranges = 58.65 to 78.93 kg

Using the examples above compute the following questions:

Hamwi Imperial Predictions

1. A male who is 5 feet 11 inches tall
2. A female who is 5 feet 5.5 inches tall
3. A male who is 5 feet 10.5 inches tall
4. A female who is 5 feet 5 inches tall
5. A female who is 5 feet 7 inches tall

Hamwi Metric Predictions

6. A male who is 168 cm tall
7. A male who is 174 cm tall
8. A female who is 159 cm tall
9. A female who is 160.4 cm tall
10. A male who is 173.2 cm tall

WHO predictions

11. A female who is 1.58 m tall
12. A male who is 175 cm tall
13. A female who is 160 cm tall
14. A male who is 1.69 m tall
15. A female who is 162 cm tall

See answers on *page 50 and 51.*

References

Kammerer, M. R., Porter, M. M., Beekley, A. C., & Tichansky, D. S. (2015). Ideal body weight calculation in the bariatric surgical population. *Journal of Gastrointestinal Surgery*, 19(10), 1758-1762.

Müller, M. J. (2016). Ideal body weight or BMI: so, what's it to be?. *The American Journal of Clinical Nutrition*, 103(5), 1193-1194

Peterson, C. M., Thomas, D. M., Blackburn, G. L., & Heymsfield, S. B. (2016). Universal equation for estimating ideal body weight and body weight at any BMI. *The American Journal of Clinical Nutrition*, *103*(5), 1197-1203.

Answer Sheet
Chapter 1

1. A man, height 1.60m, weight 70kg
   (ANS)- 27.34 kg/m^2, overweight
2. A woman, height 1.52m, weight 50kg
   (ANS)- 21.65 kg/m^2, Normal weight
3. A woman, height 1.55m, weight 48kg
   (ANS)- 20 kg/m^2, Normal weight
4. A woman, height 1.63m, weight 100kg
   (ANS)- 37.45 kg/m^2, Obese Class 2
5. A man, height 1.78m, weight 93kg
   (ANS)- 29.34 kg/m^2, overweight
6. A man, height 1.63m, weight 54kg
   (ANS)- 20.30 kg/m^2, Normal weight
7. A man, height 1.80m, weight 113kg
   (ANS)- 34.88 kg/m^2, Obese Class 1
8. A woman, height 1.65m, weight 49kg
   (ANS)- 18.01 kg/m^2, Underweight
9. A woman, height 1.52m, weight 97kg
   (ANS)- 41.99 kg/m^2, Obese Class 3
10. A man, height 1.83m, weight 61kg
    (ANS)- 18.21 kg/m^2, underweight
11. A man, height 5 feet 8 inches, weight 155 lbs
    (ANS)- 23.57 lbs/in^2, Normal weight
12. A woman, height 5 feet 4 inches, weight 130 lbs
    (ANS)- 22.31 lbs/ in^2, Normal weight
13. A woman, height 5 feet 7.5 inches, weight 147 lbs
    (ANS)- 22.68 lbs/ in^2, Normal weight
14. A woman, height 5 feet 3 inches, weight 128 lbs
    (ANS)- 22.67 lbs/ in^2, Normal weight

Chapter 1

15. A man, height 5 feet 9 inches, weight 162 lbs
    (ANS)- 23.92 lbs/ in^2, Normal weight
16. A man, height 5 feet 8 inches, weight 154 lbs
    (ANS)- 23.41 lbs/ in^2, Normal weight
17. A man, height 5 feet 8.5 inches, weight 120 lbs
    (ANS)- 17.98 lbs/ in^2, Underweight
18. A woman, height 5 feet 5 inches, weight 138 lbs
    (ANS)- 22.96 lbs/ in^2, Normal weight
19. A woman, height 5 feet 6 inches, weight 144 lbs
    (ANS)- 23.24 lbs/ in^2, Normal weight
20. A man, height 5 feet 10 inches, weight 167 lbs
    (ANS)- 23.96 lbs/ in^2, Normal weight

Chapter 2

1. 21 year old female weighs 52 kg, and is 128 cm tall. Calculate her BMR. **Ans: 1285.9 kcal**
2. 23 year old male weighs 65 kg, and is 1.63 m tall. Calculate his BMR. **Ans: 1615.1 kcal**
3. 37 year old female weighs 48 kg, and is 132 cm tall. Calculate her BMR. **Ans: 1179.5 kcal**
4. 43 year old male weighs 69 kg, and is 1.58 m tall. Calculate his BMR. **Ans: 1508.9 kcal**
5. 30 year old female weighs 54 kg, and is 1.4 m tall. Calculate her BMR. **Ans: 1284.4 kcal**
6. 33 year old male weighs 74 kg, and is 1.68 m tall. Calculate his BMR. **Ans: 1695.4 kcal**
7. 35 year old female weighs 50 kg, and is 125 cm tall. Calculate her BMR. **Ans: 1195.5 kcal**

Chapter 2

8. 27 year old male weighs 55 kg, and is 1.58 m tall. Calculate his BMR. **Ans: 1425.9 kcal**
9. 24 year old female weighs 43 kg, and is 118 cm tall. Calculate her BMR. **Ans: 1167.4 kcal**
10. 50 year old male weighs 66 kg, and is 1.61 m tall. Calculate his BMR. **Ans: 1435.2 kcal**

Chapter 3

1. What is the PAL of an individual who has total energy expenditure for the last 24 hours is 1850 Kcal and her BMR is 1480 Kcal? Categorise the person's PAL. **Ans: 1.25, sedentary**
2. What is the PAL of an individual who has total energy expenditure for the last 24 hours is 1920 Kcal and her BMR is 1525 Kcal? Categorise the person's PAL. **Ans: 1.26, sedentary**

3. What is the PAL of an individual who has total energy expenditure for the last 24 hours is 1657.5 Kcal and her BMR is 1336.5 Kcal? Categorise the person's PAL. **Ans: 1.24, sedentary**

4. What is the PAL of an individual who has total energy expenditure for the last 24 hours is 2268 Kcal and her BMR is 1748.2 Kcal? Categorise the person's PAL. **Ans: 1.30, sedentary**

Chapter 3

5. What is the PAL of an individual who has total energy expenditure for the last 24 hours is 2300 Kcal and her BMR is 1689 Kcal? Categorise the person's PAL.
Ans: 1.36, sedentary

6. What is the PAL of an individual who has total energy expenditure for the last 24 hours is 1961 Kcal and her BMR is 1265 Kcal? Categorise the person's PAL.
Ans: 1.55, moderately active

7. What is the PAL of an individual who has total energy expenditure for the last 24 hours is 1960 Kcal and her BMR is 1400 Kcal? Categorise the person's PAL.
Ans: 1.40, lightly active

8. What is the PAL of an individual who has total energy expenditure for the last 24 hours is 2250 Kcal and her BMR is 1410 Kcal? Categorise the person's PAL.
Ans: 1.60, moderately active

9. What is the PAL of an individual who has total energy expenditure for the last 24 hours is 1800 Kcal and her BMR is 1280 Kcal? Categorise the person's PAL.
Ans: 1.41, moderately active

10. What is the PAL of an individual who has total energy expenditure for the last 24 hours is 1750 Kcal and her BMR is 1400 Kcal? Categorise the person's PAL.
Ans: 1.25, moderately active

Chapter 4

1. A client consumes a juice box with 1.5 servings as the total content. Each serving contains 22 g of carbohydrates; and 16 g of protein consumed. What is the client's TEI? **Ans: 228 Kcal**

2. What is the TEI of food with the following macronutrient composition: 5 g alcohol; 12.5 g carbohydrate; 17 g protein and 3g fat? **Ans: 180 Kcal**

3. How much energy does an individual receive if he consumes 3.5 servings of a product which has 28 g of carbohydrate, 14 g of fat and 18.5 g of protein per serving? **Ans: 1092 Kcal**

4. Determine the TEI of a client who drinks 600 mls of a product that reads 250 mls per serving which has 10 g alcohol, 7 g carbohydrate and 30 g of protein per serving. **Ans: 523.2 Kcal**

5. What is the energy contribution of a product that has 15g of carbohydrate, 8 grams of protein and 4 grams of fat per serving if the client has 5 servings? **Ans: 580 Kcal**

6. What is the energy contribution of a product that has 13 g of carbohydrate, 64 g of protein and 8 g of fat, if a client has 2 servings? **Ans: 760 Kcal**

Chapter 4

7. A client consumes a 750 ml bottle of a beverage which reads 300 mls per serving. It has 40 g Carbs, 12 g fat and 28 g of alcohol per serving. What is the TEI of the client who consumes this beverage?
Ans: 1010 Kcal

8. What is the total energy in food with the following macronutrient composition: 30 g carbohydrate, 17 g protein and 5 g of fat? **Ans: 233 Kcal**

9. How much energy does a client receive from 4 servings of a product which has 11.5 g of carbohydrate, 14 g of protein and 10 g of fat?
Ans: 768 Kcal

10. Determine the total energy a client receives if he consumes 2.5 servings of a product which has 15 g of carbohydrates, 32 g of protein and 16 g fat.
Ans: 830 Kcal

Chapter 5

1. A client weighed 52kg last month and now weighs 49.5 kg. He is 1.61 m tall. He has had little intake for the 2 days. Calculate his MUST score and classify him. **Ans: MUST Score 1, medium risk; observe**

2. A client weighed 63 kg last month and now weighs 64.3 kg. He is 166 cm tall. He has had no intake for the 6 days. Calculate his MUST score and classify him. **Ans: MUST Score 2, high risk; treat**

3. A client weighed 48 kg last month and now weighs 46.2 kg. He is 1.58 m tall. He has had little intake for the 4 days. Calculate his MUST score and classify him. **Ans: MUST Score 2, high risk; treat**

4. A client weighed 61 kg last month and now weighs 60.4 kg. He is 1.75 m tall. He has had little intake for the 3 days. Calculate his MUST score and classify him. **Ans: MUST Score 1, medium risk; observe**

5. A client weighed 55kg last month and now weighs 52.6 kg. He is 163.5 cm tall. He has had little intake for the 4 days. Calculate his MUST score and classify him. **Ans: MUST Score 1, medium risk; observe**

Chapter 5

6. A client weighed 60 kg last month and now weighs 57 kg. He is 1.65 m tall. He has had little intake for the 1 day. Calculate his MUST score and classify him. **Ans: MUST Score 1, medium risk; observe**

7. A client weighed 65kg last month and now weighs 63.5 kg. He is 172 cm tall. He has had little intake for the 3 days. Calculate his MUST score and classify him. **Ans: MUST Score 0, low risk; routine clinical care**

8. A client weighed 68kg last month and now weighs 66.5 kg. He is 1.73 m tall. He has had little intake for the 6 days. Calculate his MUST score and classify him. **Ans: MUST Score 2, high risk; treat**

9. A client weighed 55kg last month and now weighs 53 kg. He is 162 cm tall. He has had little intake for the 2 days. Calculate his MUST score and classify him. **Ans: MUST Score 0, low risk; routine clinical care**

10. A client weighed 48kg last month and now weighs 47 kg. He is 158 cm tall. He has had little intake for the 4 days. Calculate his MUST score and classify him. **Ans: MUST Score 1, medium risk; observe**

Chapter 6

1. A client has a waist circumference of 71 cm and a hip circumference of 34 inches. What is **her** WHR and WHO recommendations for her?
   Ans: 0.82, Low CVD risk
2. A client has a waist circumference of 74 cm and a hip circumference of 36.8 cm. What is **her** WHR and WHO recommendations for her?
   Ans: 0.79, Low CVD risk
3. A client a waist circumference of 35 inches and a hip circumference of 33 inches. What is **his** WHR and WHO recommendations for her?
   Ans: 1.06, Increased CVD risk
4. A client a waist circumference of 34 inches and a hip circumference of 35.2 inches. What is her WHR and WHO recommendations for **her**?
   Ans: 0.96, Increased CVD risk
5. A client a waist circumference of 42 inches and a hip circumference of 46 inches. What is her WHR and WHO recommendations for **his**?
   Ans: 0.91, Increased CVD risk
6. A client a waist circumference of 79 cm and a hip circumference of 83 cm. What is her WHR and WHO recommendations for **her**?
   Ans: 0.95, Increased CVD risk
7. A client a waist circumference of 73 cm and a hip circumference of 38.2 inches. What is her WHR and WHO recommendations for **his**?
   Ans: 0.75, Low CVD risk

Chapter 6

8. A client a waist circumference of 38 inches and a hip circumference of 39.2 cm. What is her WHR and WHO recommendations for **her**?
   Ans: 0.97, Increased CVD risk
9. A client a waist circumference of 42 inches and a hip circumference of 46 inches. What is her WHR and WHO recommendations for **his**?
   Ans: 0.91, Increased CVD risk
10. A client a waist circumference of 70 cm and a hip circumference of 81 cm. What is her WHR and WHO recommendations for **her**?
    Ans: 0.86, Increased CVD risk

Chapter 7

1. Compute the energy contribution for a client who received 1350 mls of 25% DW in 24 hours.
   Ans: 1147.5 Kcal
2. Compute the energy contribution for a client who received 1800 mls of 10% DW in 24 hours.
   Ans: 612 Kcal
3. Compute the energy contribution for a client who received 2200 mls of 5% DW in 24 hours.
   Ans: 374 Kcal
4. Compute the energy contribution for a client who received 3500 mls of 10% DW in 24 hours.
   Ans: 1190 Kcal

Chapter 7

5. Compute the energy contribution for a client who received 2100 mls of 20% DW in 24 hours.
   Ans: 1428 Kcal
6. Compute the energy contribution for a client who received 1750 mls of 10% DW in 24 hours.
   Ans: 595 Kcal
7. Compute the energy contribution for a client who received 3200 mls of 5% DW in 24 hours.
   Ans: 544 Kcal
8. Compute the energy contribution for a client who received 1950 mls of 25% DW in 24 hours.
   Ans: 1657.5 Kcal
9. Compute the energy contribution for a client who received 1850 mls of 5% DW in 24 hours.
   Ans: 314.5 Kcal
10. Compute the energy contribution for a client who received 950 mls of 50% DW in 24 hours.
    Ans: 1615 Kcal

Chapter 8

Hamwi Imperial Predictions

1. A male who is 5 feet 11 inches tall
   Ans: 154.8 to 189.2 lbs
2. A female who is 5 feet 5.5 inches tall
   Ans: 114.75 to 140.25 lbs
3. A male who is 5 feet 10.5 inches tall
   Ans: 152.1 to 185.9 lbs

Chapter 8

Hamwi Imperial Predictions

4. A female who is 5 feet 5 inches tall
   Ans: 112.5 to 137.5 lbs
5. A female who is 5 feet 7 inches tall
   Ans: 121.5 to 147.5 lbs

Hamwi Metric Predictions

6. A male who is 168 cm tall **Ans: 58.64 to 71.68 kg**
7. A male who is 174 cm tall **Ans: 64.58 to 78.94 kg**
8. A female who is 159 cm tall **Ans: 45.85 to 56.03 kg**
9. A female who is 160.4 cm tall **Ans: 46.98 to 57.42 kg**
10. A male who is 173.2 cm tall **Ans: 63.79 to 77.97 kg**

WHO predictions

11. A female who is 1.58 m tall **Ans: 46.25 to 62.25 kg**
12. A male who is 175 cm tall **Ans: 56.61 to 76.19 kg**
13. A female who is 160 cm tall **Ans: 47.36 to 63.74 kg**
14. A male who is 1.69 m tall **Ans: 52.91 to 71.21 kg**
15. A female who is 162 cm tall **Ans: 48.47 to 65.24 kg**